MEDITERRANEAN FREEZER

MEALS COOKBOOK

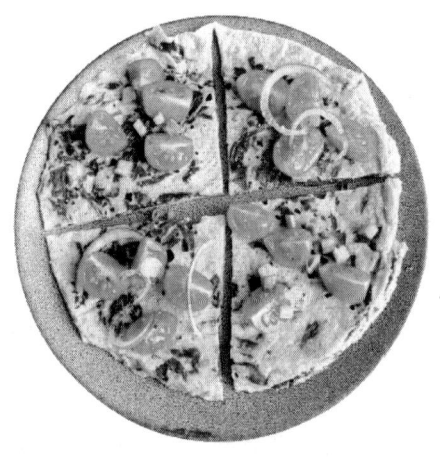

"30 Nutritious Recipes for a Mediterranean

Freezer Diet"

REGINA ANDERSON

Copyright © 2023 by Regina Anderson

DISCLAIMER

This cookbook is intended to provide general information and recipes.

The recipes provided in this cookbook are not intended to replace or be a substitute for medical advice from a physician.

The reader should consult a healthcare professional for any specific medical advice, diagnosis or treatment.

Any specific dietary advice provided in this cookbook is not intended to replace or be a substitute for medical advice from a physician.

The author is not responsible or liable for any adverse effects experienced by readers of this cookbook as a result of following the recipes or dietary advice provided.

The author makes no representations or warranties of any kind (express or implied) as to the accuracy, completeness, reliability or suitability of the recipes provided in this cookbook.

The author disclaims any and all liability for any damages arising out of the use or misuse of the recipes provided in this cookbook. The reader must also take care to ensure that the recipes provided in this cookbook are prepared and cooked safely.

The recipes provided in this cookbook are for informational purposes only and should not be used as a substitute for professional medical advice, diagnosis or treatment.

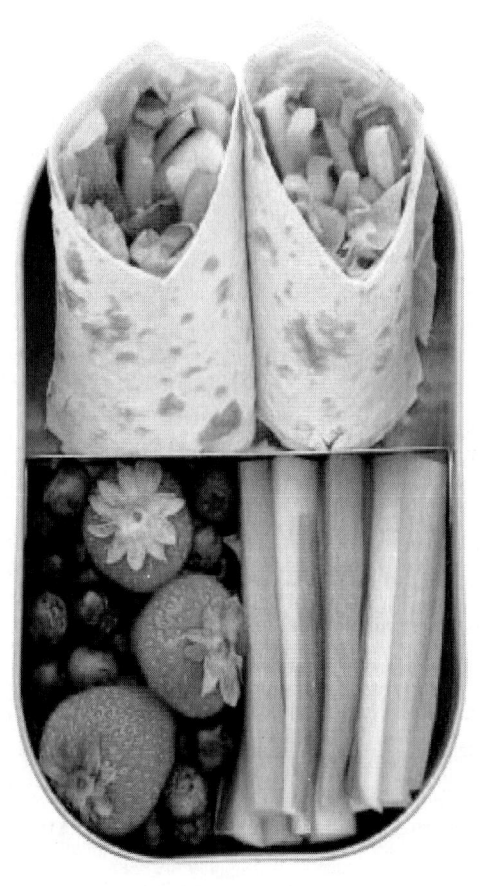

TABLE OF CONTENTS

INTRODUCTION 7

CHAPTER 1 9

UNDERSTANDING THE BASICS OF FREEZER MEALS 9

BENEFITS OF FREEZER MEALS 9

FREEZER AND REFRIGERATOR GUIDELINES 11

FREEZER TIPS AND TECHNIQUES 13

REHEATING AND THAWING GUIDELINES 15

CHAPTER 2 17

WHAT TO DO AND WHAT NOT TO DO WHEN REHEATING AND
THAWING 17

WHAT TO DO 17

WHAT NOT TO DO 20

CHAPTER 3 23

TIPS AND TRICKS FOR LABELING AND ORGANIZATION FOR
FREEZER MEALS 23

CHAPTER 4 25

14-DAY MEAL PLAN 25

CHAPTER 3 29

NUTRITIOUS RECIPES FOR A MEDITERRANEAN FREEZER MEALS
.... 29

BREAKFAST 29

Mediterranean Frittata with Spinach and Feta 29

Greek Yogurt Parfait with Fresh Berries 31

Vegetable and Hummus Breakfast Wrap 33

Quinoa Breakfast Bowl 35

Smoked Salmon and Avocado Toast 37

Mediterranean Omelet with Tomatoes and Olives 39

Olive Oil and Herb Baked Eggs 40

Chickpeas Salad 42

Greek Yogurt Smoothie with Banana and Almonds 44

Whole Wheat Mediterranean Breakfast Burrito 46

LUNCH 48

Lemon Herb Baked Salmon with Roasted Vegetables................................ 48

Lentil and Vegetable Moussaka 51

Shrimp and Feta Orzo Salad.. 54

Grilled Eggplant and Hummus Wrap 55

Tomato and Basil Bruschetta with Grilled Chicken.................................... 58

Spinach and Feta Stuffed Bell Peppers... 60

Greek Salad with Grilled Chicken.. 62

Mediterranean Turkey and Vegetable Skewers... 65

Baked Zucchini and Tomato Casserole.. 67

Olive and Herb Crusted Cod with Quinoa.. 69

DINNER... 72

Baked Mediterranean Chicken with Lemon and Olives 72

Lemon Herb Quinoa with Roasted Vegetables 74

Mediterranean Shrimp and Tomato Skewers 76

Greek Lamb Meatballs with Mint Yogurt Sauce 78

Roasted Eggplant and Chickpea Stew 81

Tomato Basil Cod Fillets 83

Mediterranean Turkey and Zucchini Patties 85

Quinoa Tabbouleh with Cucumber and Cherry Tomatoes 88

Greek Style Stuffed Peppers with Ground Turkey...................................... 91

Chickpea and Spinach Curry with Couscous... 94

CONCLUSION 97

INTRODUCTION

Mediterranean freezer meals are a quick and health-conscious way to prepare meals that are based on the region's incredibly varied and nourishing food.

Mediterranean cuisine, renowned for its heart-healthy ingredients and exquisite taste, is now more accessible and convenient than ever with the introduction of Mediterranean freezer meals.

In the fast-paced rhythm of modern life, finding the time to prepare nutritious and delicious meals can be a challenge.

Whether you're a seasoned home chef or someone looking to simplify their meal preparation, these freezer meals offer a delightful escape to the sun-soaked shores of the Mediterranean without sacrificing taste or nutrition.

Imagine savoring the bold aromas of garlic, olive oil, and fragrant herbs as you indulge in dishes inspired by the coastal cuisines of Greece, Italy, Spain, and beyond.

From succulent grilled meats to aromatic vegetable stews, these freezer meals capture the essence of the Mediterranean diet, known for its emphasis on fresh produce, lean proteins, and heart-healthy fats.

Finally, the beauty of Mediterranean freezer meals lies in their versatility and ease of preparation. Now, go ahead and explore the recipes provided in this book and have fun while at it.

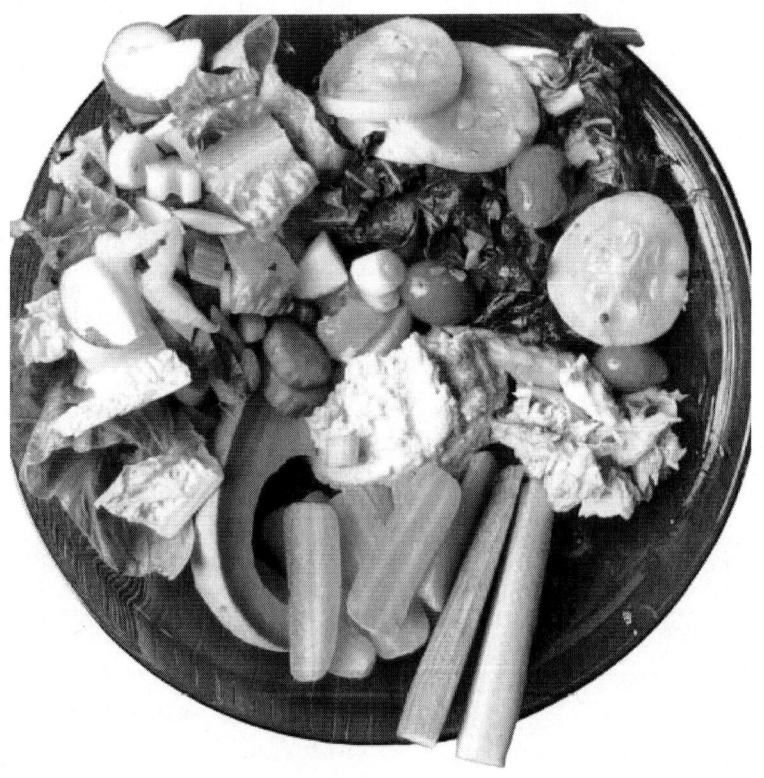

CHAPTER 1

UNDERSTANDING THE BASICS OF FREEZER MEALS

BENEFITS OF FREEZER MEALS

1. **Time-Saving Convenience:** Freezer meals allow you to invest time upfront in preparing and cooking meals, saving you precious time on busy weeknights or during hectic periods.

2. **Batch Cooking Efficiency:** Prepare large quantities of meals at once, enabling you to take advantage of bulk ingredients and streamline your cooking process.

3. **Reduced Food Waste:** By freezing meals in portions, you can reduce the risk of food spoilage and waste, as you only thaw and heat what you need.

4. **Cost-Effective Planning:** Buying ingredients in bulk for freezer meals often results in cost savings, making it an economical choice for budget-conscious individuals or families.

5. **Preservation of Nutrients:** Freezing meals at their peak freshness helps retain essential nutrients, ensuring that your meals are not only convenient but also nutritionally valuable.

6. **Long-Term Meal Planning:** With freezer meals, you can plan for the long term, stocking your freezer with a variety of dishes that can be enjoyed over an extended period.

7. **Healthier Eating Choices:** Preparing freezer meals allows you to control the ingredients, making it easier to opt for healthier choices and adhere to dietary restrictions.

8. **Variety and Versatility:** Freeze a diverse range of meals to ensure variety in your diet, preventing mealtime monotony and keeping your taste buds satisfied.

9. **Portion Control:** Freezer meals can be portioned according to your dietary needs, aiding in portion control and preventing overeating.

10. **Flexible Cooking Schedule:** Freezer meals offer flexibility, allowing you to cook and freeze when it's convenient for

FREEZER AND REFRIGERATOR GUIDELINES

1. **Proper Temperature Settings for freezer:** Maintain a temperature of 0°F (-18°C) or lower to ensure the safe storage of frozen foods.

2. **Proper Temperature Settings for refrigerator:** Keep the refrigerator at 40°F (4°C) or below to slow down bacterial growth.

3. **Organization is Key:** Arrange items in the freezer and refrigerator logically for easy access and to prevent food from getting lost or overlooked.

4. **Labeling and Dating:** Clearly label and date all items stored in the freezer to track freshness and avoid consuming items past their prime.

5. **Airtight Packaging:** Use airtight, moisture-resistant packaging to prevent freezer burn and maintain the quality of frozen foods.

6. **Avoid Overcrowding:** Allow air to circulate freely in the freezer and refrigerator to maintain even temperatures. Overcrowding can lead to uneven cooling.

7. **Thawing Safely:** Thaw frozen items in the refrigerator, in cold water, or using the microwave to ensure a safe and controlled thawing process.

8. **Temperature Monitoring:** Regularly check the freezer and refrigerator temperatures with a thermometer to ensure they stay within the recommended ranges.

9. **First In, First Out (FIFO):** Practice the FIFO method when organizing the freezer and refrigerator, using older items before newer ones to minimize food waste.

10. **Proper Storage for Fresh Produce:** Store fruits and vegetables in designated crisper drawers in the refrigerator to maintain optimal humidity levels and freshness.

11. **Safe Thawing Practices:** Thaw meat and poultry on a plate or in a container to prevent juices from contaminating other foods in the refrigerator.

12. **Maintain Cleanliness:** Regularly clean the freezer and refrigerator, removing any spills or expired items to prevent the growth of bacteria and odors.

FREEZER TIPS AND TECHNIQUES

1. **Flash Freezing:** Spread items like berries or diced vegetables on a tray and freeze them individually before transferring to a container. This prevents them from clumping together, making it easier to use only the desired amount.

2. **Vacuum Sealing:** Use a vacuum sealer to remove air from packaging, reducing the risk of freezer burn and prolonging the shelf life of frozen items.

3. **Double Wrapping:** Place an additional layer of plastic wrap or aluminum foil around items already in freezer bags to add an extra barrier against freezer burn.

4. **Freeze in Portions:** Portion meals before freezing to make it simple to thaw and reheat exactly what you need, reducing waste.

5. **Labeling with Instructions:** Clearly label packages with the item name, date of freezing, and any reheating instructions to make meal preparation more straightforward.

6. **Ice Cube Trays for Sauces:** Freeze small portions of sauces, broth, or pesto in ice cube trays. Once frozen,

transfer the cubes to a labeled bag for easy portioning.

7. **Bread Slicing Before Freezing:** Slice bread before freezing so you can easily take out individual slices without having to thaw the entire loaf.

8. **Shelf Organization:** Arrange items in the freezer by category, placing similar items together. This makes it easier to locate specific items and prevents the freezer from becoming overly cluttered.

9. **Use Freezer-Friendly Containers:** Invest in containers specifically designed for freezing to prevent freezer burn and protect the quality of your food.

10. **Layering with Parchment Paper:** Place a layer of parchment paper between items like pancakes or burgers before freezing to prevent them from sticking together.

11. **Pre-Cook and Freeze:** Cook large batches of meals and freeze individual portions for quick and easy reheating on busy days.

REHEATING AND THAWING GUIDELINES

1. For large items like casseroles or roasts, consider reheating in stages, starting at a lower temperature to ensure the entire dish is evenly heated without overcooking the outer layers.

2. Thaw frozen items in the refrigerator to maintain a safe temperature and minimize the risk of bacterial growth. This method allows for controlled and even thawing.

3. Use the microwave for quick thawing of smaller items, but be sure to follow the appliance's guidelines and cook the food immediately after thawing.

4. Submerge sealed packages in cold water for faster thawing. Change the water every 30 minutes to ensure a consistent temperature.

5. When thawing in the refrigerator, keep items in their original packaging to prevent cross-contamination and preserve moisture.

6. Use the defrost setting on your microwave for more controlled thawing. Monitor the process closely to avoid partial cooking.

7. Ensure that reheated foods reach a safe internal temperature of at least 165°F (74°C) to eliminate any potential bacteria and ensure food safety.

8. Stir soups, stews, and other liquid-based dishes while reheating to promote even distribution of heat and prevent hot spots.

9. Cover dishes with a lid, microwave-safe cover, or damp paper towel when reheating to retain moisture and prevent drying out.

10. Thaw meats separately from other items to avoid cross-contamination. Place meat on a plate or in a sealed bag to catch any juices.

11. Reheat large quantities of food in smaller portions to ensure even heating and maintain the quality of the entire batch.

12. When reheating items like casseroles or baked goods, consider using the oven for more even heating and to retain texture.

13. Some foods, like salads or delicate greens, may not reheat well. Consider eating these items fresh rather than attempting to reheat them.

CHAPTER 2

WHAT TO DO AND WHAT NOT TO DO WHEN REHEATING AND THAWING

WHAT TO DO

When reheating and thawing, it's crucial to follow proper guidelines to ensure food safety and maintain the quality of your meals. Here's what you should do:

1. **Check Temperature Guidelines:** Ensure that you're reheating food to a safe internal temperature, typically 165°F (74°C) for most dishes. Use a food thermometer to verify the temperature.

2. **Reheat in Portions:** Reheat larger quantities of food in smaller portions to ensure even heating and avoid undercooked or overcooked sections.

3. **Use Microwave Safely:** Follow the manufacturer's instructions for your microwave, and use the appropriate settings for reheating. Stir or rotate the food during the process to promote even heating.

4. **Cover for Moisture Retention:** Cover dishes with a lid, microwave-safe cover, or damp paper towel to

retain moisture and prevent drying out during the reheating process.

5. **Stirring:** Stir soups, stews, and other liquid-based dishes during reheating to distribute heat evenly and avoid hot spots.

6. **Oven Reheating:** Consider using the oven for reheating larger items or baked goods, as it provides more even heating and helps maintain texture.

7. **Avoid Reheating Certain Foods:** Some foods, like salads or delicate greens, may not reheat well. Plan your meals to minimize the need for reheating such items.

8. **Reheat Immediately:** Reheat food immediately after thawing to minimize the time it spends at temperatures conducive to bacterial growth.

9. **Refrigerator Thawing:** Thaw frozen items in the refrigerator to maintain a safe and controlled temperature. This is the safest method for most foods.

10. **Microwave Thawing:** Use the microwave for quick thawing of smaller items. Follow the microwave's

guidelines and cook the food immediately after thawing.

11. **Cold Water Thawing:** Submerge sealed packages in cold water, changing the water every 30 minutes. This method is faster than refrigerator thawing but requires more attention.

12. **Thaw in Original Packaging:** Thaw items in their original packaging when using the refrigerator method to preserve moisture and prevent cross-contamination.

13. **Defrost Setting:** Use the defrost setting on your microwave for controlled thawing. Monitor the process closely to prevent partial cooking.

14. **Thaw Meats Separately:** Thaw meats on a plate or in a sealed bag to catch any juices and prevent cross-contamination with other foods.

15. **Plan Ahead:** Plan your meals to allow sufficient time for proper thawing. Avoid rushing the process to ensure safety and quality.

WHAT NOT TO DO

1. **Don't Thaw at Room Temperature:** Avoid thawing frozen food at room temperature, as this can lead to bacterial growth. Use methods like the refrigerator, microwave, or cold water instead.

2. **Don't Thaw and Refreeze:** Once food has been thawed, avoid refreezing it, as this can compromise the texture, flavor, and safety of the item.

3. **Don't Thaw on the Counter Overnight:** Leaving food to thaw on the counter overnight is a food safety risk, as it allows bacteria to multiply rapidly in the temperature danger zone.

4. **Avoid Thawing in Hot Water:** Do not use hot water for thawing, as it can cause uneven thawing and may promote bacterial growth.

5. **Avoid Thawing in Microwave Without Rotation:** If using a microwave for thawing, avoid simply setting it and forgetting it. Rotate and turn the item during the process to ensure even thawing.

6. **Don't Reheat in Large Chunks:** When reheating large dishes, avoid doing so in one big chunk, as this

can result in uneven heating. Reheat in smaller portions for better results.

7. **Avoid Reheating Fried Foods in the Microwave:** Fried foods tend to lose their crispiness when reheated in the microwave. Use an oven or toaster oven for better results.

8. **Don't Overcrowd the Microwave:** When reheating multiple items in the microwave, avoid overcrowding the turntable. This ensures that each item is heated evenly.

9. **Avoid Leaving Food Unattended During Reheating:** Do not leave food unattended while reheating, especially in the microwave, to prevent overcooking or burning.

10. **Don't Reheat Certain Foods:** Some foods, like eggs in their shells or whole fruits, can explode when reheated. Avoid reheating these items.

11. **Avoid Using Non-Microwave Safe Containers:** Do not use containers that are not labeled as microwave-safe for reheating in the microwave, as they may release harmful chemicals.

12. **Don't Reheat Seafood in a Closed Space:** Avoid reheating seafood in an enclosed space, such as an office microwave, as the strong aroma may be unpleasant to others.

13. **Avoid Rapid Temperature Changes:** Avoid exposing frozen items to rapid temperature changes, such as moving them from the freezer to a hot oven. Gradual thawing is safer and helps maintain food quality.

14. **Don't Assume All Foods Reheat the Same Way:** Different foods require different reheating methods. Don't assume that one method fits all; follow specific guidelines for each type of food.

15. **Avoid Thawing and Reheating for Extended Periods:** Don't leave thawed or reheated food at room temperature for extended periods. Consume or refrigerate promptly to prevent bacterial growth.

CHAPTER 3

TIPS AND TRICKS FOR LABELING AND ORGANIZATION FOR FREEZER MEALS

1. **Label Before Freezing:** Label containers or bags before filling them to avoid confusion and ensure accurate information is recorded.

2. **Color-Coding:** Assign specific colors to different categories of meals or types of proteins. For example, use one color for chicken dishes and another for vegetarian options.

3. **Use Waterproof Ink:** Write labels with waterproof ink or use waterproof labels to prevent smudging or fading when condensation occurs in the freezer.

4. **Include Ingredients:** Note key ingredients or allergens on the label for quick reference, especially if you're preparing meals for others with specific dietary needs.

5. **Reusable Labels:** Consider using reusable labels that can be easily wiped clean and rewritten, saving both time and resources.

6. **Label on Lids:** If using containers with lids, label both the container and the lid to ensure information remains visible regardless of how the container is stacked.

7. **Shelf Labels:** Label shelves in your freezer to designate specific areas for different types of meals, making it easier to locate items quickly.

8. **Inventory Rotation:** Keep track of what's in your freezer and rotate items to ensure older meals are used first, reducing the risk of food waste.

9. **Use Freezer Tape:** Consider using freezer tape for labeling, as it adheres well in cold temperatures and can be easily removed without leaving sticky residue.

10. **Label Portions:** If you've portioned meals before freezing, label the quantity on the container or bag to know how much is in each serving.

11. **Group Similar Items:** Group similar items together, such as soups or casseroles, to create designated sections in your freezer for easy navigation.

CHAPTER 4

14-DAY MEAL PLAN

DAY 1

Breakfast: Mediterranean Frittata with Spinach and Feta

Lunch: Lemon Herb Baked Salmon with Roasted Vegetables

Dinner: Baked Mediterranean Chicken with Lemon and Olives

DAY 2

Breakfast: Greek Yogurt Parfait with Fresh Berries

Lunch: Lentil and Vegetable Moussaka

Dinner: Lemon Herb Quinoa with Roasted Vegetables

DAY 3

Breakfast: Vegetable and Hummus Breakfast Wrap

Lunch: Shrimp and Feta Orzo Salad

Dinner: Mediterranean Shrimp and Tomato Skewers

DAY 4

Breakfast: Quinoa Breakfast Bowl

Lunch: Grilled Eggplant and Hummus Wrap

Dinner: Greek Lamb Meatballs with Mint Yogurt Sauce

DAY 5

Breakfast: Smoked Salmon and Avocado Toast

Lunch: Tomato and Basil Bruschetta with Grilled Chicken

Dinner: Roasted Eggplant and Chickpea Stew

DAY 6

Breakfast: Mediterranean Omelet with Tomatoes and Olives

Lunch: Spinach and Feta Stuffed Bell Peppers

Dinner: Tomato Basil Cod Fillets

DAY 7

Breakfast: Olive Oil and Herb Baked Eggs

Lunch: Greek Salad with Grilled Chicken

Dinner: Mediterranean Turkey and Zucchini Patties

DAY 8

Breakfast: Chickpeas Salad

Lunch: Mediterranean Turkey and Vegetable Skewers

Dinner: Quinoa Tabbouleh with Cucumber and Cherry Tomatoes

DAY 9

Breakfast: Greek Yogurt Smoothie with Banana and Almonds

Lunch: Greek Style Stuffed Peppers with Ground Turkey

Dinner: Whole Wheat Mediterranean Breakfast Burrito

DAY 10

Breakfast: Olive and Herb Crusted Cod with Quinoa

Lunch: Chickpea and Spinach Curry with Couscous

Dinner: Roasted Eggplant and Chickpea Stew

DAY 11

Breakfast: Mediterranean Frittata with Spinach and Feta

Lunch: Lemon Herb Baked Salmon with Roasted Vegetables

Dinner: Baked Mediterranean Chicken with Lemon and Olives

DAY 12

Breakfast: Greek Yogurt Parfait with Fresh Berries

Lunch: Lentil and Vegetable Moussaka

Dinner: Lemon Herb Quinoa with Roasted Vegetables

DAY 13

Breakfast: Vegetable and Hummus Breakfast Wrap

Lunch: Shrimp and Feta Orzo Salad

Dinner: Mediterranean Shrimp and Tomato Skewers

DAY 14

Breakfast: Quinoa Breakfast Bowl

Lunch: Grilled Eggplant and Hummus Wrap

Dinner: Greek Lamb Meatballs with Mint Yogurt Sauce

CHAPTER 3

NUTRITIOUS RECIPES FOR A MEDITERRANEAN FREEZER MEALS

BREAKFAST

Mediterranean Frittata with Spinach and Feta

Preparation Time: 30 minutes

Serves: 4

Calories: 200 **Sugar:** 1g **Sodium:** 300mg

Ingredients:

8 large eggs

1 cup fresh spinach, chopped

1/2 cup feta cheese, crumbled

1/4 cup red onion, finely chopped

2 tablespoons olive oil

Salt and pepper to taste

Method of Preparation:

1. Set the oven's temperature to 175°C/350°F.
2. Beat the eggs and add salt and pepper to taste in a bowl.
3. In a skillet that is oven safe, warm the olive oil over medium heat.
4. Add chopped spinach and simmer till wilted after sautéing red onions until they become soft.
5. Over the vegetables in the skillet, pour the beaten eggs.
6. Evenly scatter the crumbled feta on top of the eggs.
7. Simmer for two to three minutes, or until the edges are set.
8. Place the skillet in the oven that has been preheated, and bake for 15 to 20 minutes, or until the frittata is brown and set.
9. After letting it cool, cut it into wedges.

Freeze for later:

1. After cooking the meal, allow it to cool off.
2. Collect all the necessary supplies, such as; freezer-safe containers or bags, labels and a waterproof

marker, plastic wrap or aluminum foil, Freezer tape (optional) and airtight vacuum sealer (optional)

3. Divide the meals into 4 containers or bags.

4. Clearly label each container or bag with the name of the dish, date of preparation, and any reheating instructions.

5. Lay bags flat in the freezer for quicker freezing and easy stacking. For containers, leave some space at the top to accommodate expansion during freezing.

6. Use older meals before newer ones to ensure nothing goes to waste.

7. Thaw and Reheat Safely

Greek Yogurt Parfait with Fresh Berries

Preparation Time: 10 minutes

Serves: 2

Calories: 250 **Sugar:** 15g **Sodium:** 50mg

Ingredients:

2 cups Greek yogurt

1 cup mixed fresh berries (strawberries, blueberries, raspberries)

1/4 cup honey

1/2 cup granola

Method of Preparation:

1. Layer Greek yogurt into glasses or bowls for serving.
2. Place a layer of mixed, raw berries on top.
3. Pour honey on top of the berries.
4. Add granola on top for crunch.
5. Continue layering as needed.

Freeze for later:

1. After cooking the meal, allow it to cool off.
2. Collect all the necessary supplies, such as; freezer-safe containers or bags, labels and a waterproof marker, plastic wrap or aluminum foil, Freezer tape (optional) and airtight vacuum sealer (optional)
3. Divide the meals into 2 containers or bags.
4. Clearly label each container or bag with the name of the dish, date of preparation, and any reheating instructions.

5. Lay bags flat in the freezer for quicker freezing and easy stacking. For containers, leave some space at the top to accommodate expansion during freezing.

6. Use older meals before newer ones to ensure nothing goes to waste.

7. Thaw and Reheat Safely

Vegetable and Hummus Breakfast Wrap

Preparation Time: 15 minutes

Serves: 4

Calories: 300 **Sugar:** 5g **Sodium:** 400mg

Ingredients:

4 whole wheat tortillas

1 cup hummus

1 cup cherry tomatoes, halved

1 cucumber, thinly sliced

1 bell pepper, thinly sliced

1/2 red onion, thinly sliced

Fresh parsley, chopped (for garnish)

Method of Preparation:

1. On each tortilla, generously spread a layer of hummus.
2. Arrange the bell pepper, cucumber, red onion, and cherry tomatoes in layers on the tortillas.
3. For extra taste, sprinkle with finely chopped fresh parsley.
4. If necessary, firmly roll up the wraps and fasten with toothpicks.
5. To serve, cut in half diagonally.

Freeze for later:

1. After cooking the meal, allow it to cool off.
2. Collect all the necessary supplies, such as; freezer-safe containers or bags, labels and a waterproof marker, plastic wrap or aluminum foil, Freezer tape (optional) and airtight vacuum sealer (optional)
3. Divide the meals into 4 containers or bags.
4. Clearly label each container or bag with the name of the dish, date of preparation, and any reheating instructions.

5. Lay bags flat in the freezer for quicker freezing and easy stacking. For containers, leave some space at the top to accommodate expansion during freezing.

6. Use older meals before newer ones to ensure nothing goes to waste.

7. Thaw and Reheat Safely

Quinoa Breakfast Bowl

Preparation Time: 20 minutes

Serves: 2

Calories: 400-450 **Sugar:** 20g **Sodium:** 50mg

Ingredients:

1 cup quinoa

2 cups water

1 cup Greek yogurt

1 cup mixed berries (strawberries, blueberries, raspberries)

1 tablespoon honey

1/4 cup chopped nuts (almonds, walnuts)

Fresh mint leaves for garnish

Method of Preparation:

1. Wash the quinoa in cool water.

2. Put the quinoa in a pot with some water.

3. After bringing to a boil, lower the heat and simmer the quinoa for 15 minutes or until the water is absorbed.

4. Arrange cooked quinoa, Greek yogurt, chopped almonds, and mixed berries in serving bowls.

5. Add a honey drizzle and some fresh mint leaves as garnish.

Freeze for later:

1. After cooking the meal, allow it to cool off.

2. Collect all the necessary supplies, such as; freezer-safe containers or bags, labels and a waterproof marker, plastic wrap or aluminum foil, Freezer tape (optional) and airtight vacuum sealer (optional)

3. Divide the meals into 2 containers or bags.

4. Clearly label each container or bag with the name of the dish, date of preparation, and any reheating instructions.

5. Lay bags flat in the freezer for quicker freezing and easy stacking. For containers, leave some space at the top to accommodate expansion during freezing.

6. Use older meals before newer ones to ensure nothing goes to waste.

7. Thaw and Reheat Safely

Smoked Salmon and Avocado Toast

Preparation Time: 15 minutes

Serves: 2

Calories: 350-400 **Sugar:** 2g **Sodium:** 600mg

Ingredients:

2 slices whole-grain bread

1 ripe avocado

4 ounces smoked salmon

1 tablespoon capers

1 tablespoon cream cheese

Fresh dill for garnish

Lemon wedges (optional)

Method of Preparation:

1. Toast the slices of wholegrain bread.

2. Spread the mashed avocado evenly over the toasted bread.

3. Add a dollop of cream cheese, capers, and smoked salmon on the top of each slice.

4. If preferred, serve with lemon wedges and garnish with fresh dill.

Freeze for later:

1. After cooking the meal, allow it to cool off.

2. Collect all the necessary supplies, such as; freezer-safe containers or bags, labels and a waterproof marker, plastic wrap or aluminum foil, Freezer tape (optional) and airtight vacuum sealer (optional)

3. Divide the meals into 2 containers or bags.

4. Clearly label each container or bag with the name of the dish, date of preparation, and any reheating instructions.

5. Lay bags flat in the freezer for quicker freezing and easy stacking. For containers, leave some space at the top to accommodate expansion during freezing.

6. Use older meals before newer ones to ensure nothing goes to waste.

7. Thaw and Reheat Safely

Mediterranean Omelet with Tomatoes and Olives

Preparation Time: 15 minutes

Serves: 2

Calories: 300-350 **Sugar:** 2g **Sodium:** 400mg

Ingredients:

4 large eggs

1/4 cup feta cheese, crumbled

1/2 cup cherry tomatoes, halved

1/4 cup Kalamata olives, sliced

1 tablespoon olive oil

Fresh basil for garnish

Salt and pepper to taste

Method of Preparation:

1. In a bowl, whisk together eggs and add pepper and salt to taste.
2. In a skillet over medium heat, warm the olive oil.
3. Whisked eggs should be added to the skillet and given a little time to solidify.
4. Over one half of the omelet, scatter the olives, cherry tomatoes, and feta cheese.
5. Once the eggs have totally set, fold the omelet in half.

Olive Oil and Herb Baked Eggs

Preparation Time: 20 minutes

Serves: 2

Calories: 250 **Sugar:** 2g

Ingredients:

4 large eggs

2 tablespoons extra virgin olive oil

1 teaspoon dried oregano

1 teaspoon dried thyme

Salt and pepper to taste

2 tablespoons feta cheese (optional)

Fresh parsley for garnish

Method of Preparation:

1. Turn the oven on to 375°F, or 190°C.

2. Pour olive oil onto a baking dish or individual ramekins.

3. Make sure the eggs are equally spread out as you crack them into the dish.

4. Season the eggs with salt, pepper, thyme, and dried oregano.

5. Top with crumbled feta cheese.

6. Bake for 12 to 15 minutes, or until the yolks are still runny but the whites are set.

Freeze for later:

1. After cooking the meal, allow it to cool off.

2. Collect all the necessary supplies, such as; freezer-safe containers or bags, labels and a waterproof marker, plastic wrap or aluminum foil, Freezer tape (optional) and airtight vacuum sealer (optional)

3. Divide the meals into 2 containers or bags.

4. Clearly label each container or bag with the name of the dish, date of preparation, and any reheating instructions.

5. Lay bags flat in the freezer for quicker freezing and easy stacking. For containers, leave some space at the top to accommodate expansion during freezing.

6. Use older meals before newer ones to ensure nothing goes to waste.

7. Thaw and Reheat Safely

Chickpeas Salad

Preparation Time: 15 minutes

Serves: 4

Calories: 300 **Sugar:** 3g **Sodium:** 400mg

Ingredients:

2 cups canned chickpeas, drained and rinsed

1 cucumber, diced

1 cup cherry tomatoes, halved

1/2 red onion, finely chopped

1/4 cup feta cheese, crumbled

2 tablespoons extra virgin olive oil

1 tablespoon red wine vinegar

1 teaspoon dried oregano

Salt and pepper to taste

Fresh parsley for garnish

Method of Preparation:

1. Chickpeas, cucumber, cherry tomatoes, red onion, and feta cheese should all be combined in a big bowl.
2. Mix the olive oil, red wine vinegar, dried oregano, salt, and pepper in a small bowl.
3. After adding the dressing to the salad, toss to mix.
4. Before serving, place the fresh parsley garnish on top and chill for a minimum of half an hour.

Freeze for later:

1. After cooking the meal, allow it to cool off.
2. Collect all the necessary supplies, such as; freezer-safe containers or bags, labels and a waterproof marker, plastic wrap or aluminum foil, Freezer tape (optional) and airtight vacuum sealer (optional)

3. Divide the meals into 4 containers or bags.

4. Clearly label each container or bag with the name of the dish, date of preparation, and any reheating instructions.

5. Lay bags flat in the freezer for quicker freezing and easy stacking. For containers, leave some space at the top to accommodate expansion during freezing.

6. Use older meals before newer ones to ensure nothing goes to waste.

7. Thaw and Reheat Safely

Greek Yogurt Smoothie with Banana and Almonds

Preparation Time: 10 minutes

Serves: 2

Calories: 250 **Sugar:** 15g **Sodium:** 60mg

Ingredients:

1 cup Greek yogurt

1 ripe banana

1/2 cup almond milk

1/4 cup almonds, chopped

1 tablespoon honey

1/2 teaspoon vanilla extract

Ice cubes (optional)

Method of Preparation:

1. Greek yogurt, banana, almond milk, sliced almonds, honey, and vanilla essence should all be combined in a blender.
2. Blend till creamy and smooth.
3. If using ice cubes, add them and blend once more until well mixed.
4. Transfer into glasses and serve right away.

Freeze for later:

1. After preparing the meal, allow it sit for few minutes.
2. Collect all the necessary supplies, such as; freezer-safe containers or bags, labels and a waterproof marker, plastic wrap or aluminum foil, Freezer tape (optional) and airtight vacuum sealer (optional)
3. Divide the meals into 2 containers or bags.

4. Clearly label each container or bag with the name of the dish, date of preparation, and any reheating instructions.

5. Lay bags flat in the freezer for quicker freezing and easy stacking. For containers, leave some space at the top to accommodate expansion during freezing.

6. Use older meals before newer ones to ensure nothing goes to waste.

7. Thaw and Reheat Safely

Whole Wheat Mediterranean Breakfast Burrito

Preparation Time: 20 minutes

Serves: 4

Calories: 350 **Sugar:** 2g **Sodium:** 550mg

Ingredients:

4 whole wheat tortillas

4 eggs, scrambled

1 cup spinach, chopped

1 cup cherry tomatoes, diced

1/2 cup feta cheese, crumbled

1/4 cup Kalamata olives, sliced

2 tablespoons olive oil

Salt and pepper to taste

Fresh parsley for garnish

Method of Preparation:

1. Warm up some olive oil in a pan over medium heat.
2. When the spinach has wilted, add the chopped spinach and cherry tomatoes and sauté.
3. Stir the scrambled eggs in the pan until they are fully done.
4. Use a microwave or a dry skillet to reheat the tortillas.
5. Spoon some of the egg mixture onto each tortilla.
6. Add sliced Kalamata olives and crumbled feta cheese on top.
7. Add salt and pepper for seasoning, then top with fresh parsley.
8. After folding the tortilla's edges, roll it into a burrito.

Freeze for later:

1. After cooking the meal, allow it to cool off.

2. Collect all the necessary supplies, such as; freezer-safe containers or bags, labels and a waterproof marker, plastic wrap or aluminum foil, Freezer tape (optional) and airtight vacuum sealer (optional)

3. Divide the meals into 4 containers or bags.

4. Clearly label each container or bag with the name of the dish, date of preparation, and any reheating instructions.

5. Lay bags flat in the freezer for quicker freezing and easy stacking. For containers, leave some space at the top to accommodate expansion during freezing.

6. Use older meals before newer ones to ensure nothing goes to waste.

7. Thaw and Reheat Safely

LUNCH

Lemon Herb Baked Salmon with Roasted Vegetables

Preparation Time: 30 minutes

Serves: 4

Calories: 350 **Sugar:** 5g **Sodium:** 300mg

Ingredients:

4 salmon fillets

1 lemon (juiced and zested)

3 tablespoons olive oil

2 cloves garlic (minced)

1 teaspoon dried oregano

1 teaspoon dried thyme

Salt and pepper to taste

1-pound mixed vegetables (e.g., cherry tomatoes, zucchini, bell peppers)

Method of Preparation:

1. Set oven temperature to 400°F, or 200°C.
2. To make the marinade, combine the lemon zest, lemon juice, olive oil, minced garlic, dried oregano, dried thyme, salt, and pepper in a small bowl.

3. Transfer the salmon fillets to a shallow dish and cover them with half of the marinade.

4. Give it a minimum of fifteen minutes to marinate.

5. Place the mixed veggies in a baking sheet arrangement.

6. After drizzling the leftover marinade over the veggies, toss to cover.

7. Arrange the marinated salmon fillets onto the vegetable-topped baking sheet.

8. Bake for 15 to 20 minutes, or until the veggies are soft and the salmon is thoroughly cooked, in a preheated oven.

9. Before dividing the meal into individual serves, let it cool.

Freeze for later:

1. After cooking the meal, allow it to cool off.

2. Collect all the necessary supplies, such as; freezer-safe containers or bags, labels and a waterproof marker, plastic wrap or aluminum foil, Freezer tape (optional) and airtight vacuum sealer (optional)

3. Divide the meals into 4 containers or bags.

4. Clearly label each container or bag with the name of the dish, date of preparation, and any reheating instructions.

5. Lay bags flat in the freezer for quicker freezing and easy stacking. For containers, leave some space at the top to accommodate expansion during freezing.

6. Use older meals before newer ones to ensure nothing goes to waste.

7. Thaw and Reheat Safely

Lentil and Vegetable Moussaka

Preparation Time: 1 hour

Serves: 6

Calories: 400 **Sugar:** 8g **Sodium:** 450mg

Ingredients:

1 cup dry lentils

2 eggplants, sliced

1 onion, chopped

2 cloves garlic, minced

1 can (14 oz) diced tomatoes

1 teaspoon dried oregano

1 teaspoon dried thyme

1 teaspoon ground cinnamon

Salt and pepper to taste

2 cups béchamel sauce (made with milk, flour, and butter)

Method of Preparation:

1. Follow the cooking directions on the package for the lentils.
2. Turn the oven on to 375°F, or 190°C.
3. Minced garlic and diced onion should be sautéed in a pan until they become tender.
4. When the eggplant slices are golden brown, add them and continue to cook.
5. Add the chopped tomatoes, cooked lentils, ground cinnamon, dried thyme, dried oregano, and salt & pepper to taste. After ten minutes, simmer.
6. Arrange the lentil and vegetable mixture in a baking dish and cover with the béchamel sauce.

7. Bake for 30 to 40 minutes, or until the top is golden brown, in a preheated oven.

8. Let the moussaka cool completely before slicing it into serving portions.

Freeze for later:

1. After cooking the meal, allow it to cool off.

2. Collect all the necessary supplies, such as; freezer-safe containers or bags, labels and a waterproof marker, plastic wrap or aluminum foil, Freezer tape (optional) and airtight vacuum sealer (optional)

3. Divide the meals into 6 containers or bags.

4. Clearly label each container or bag with the name of the dish, date of preparation, and any reheating instructions.

5. Lay bags flat in the freezer for quicker freezing and easy stacking. For containers, leave some space at the top to accommodate expansion during freezing.

6. Use older meals before newer ones to ensure nothing goes to waste.

7. Thaw and Reheat Safely

Shrimp and Feta Orzo Salad

Preparation Time: 40 minutes

Serves: 4

Calories: 300 **Sugar:** 4g **Sodium:** 350mg

Ingredients:

1 cup orzo pasta

1 pound shrimp, peeled and deveined

1 cup cherry tomatoes, halved

1 cucumber, diced

1/2 cup Kalamata olives, sliced

1/2 cup crumbled feta cheese

2 tablespoons olive oil

2 tablespoons red wine vinegar

1 teaspoon dried oregano

Salt and pepper to taste

Method of Preparation:

1. Follow the directions on the package to cook the orzo pasta. Empty and allow it to cool.
2. Cook the shrimp in a pan until they become opaque and pink.
3. Cooked orzo, cooked shrimp, chopped cucumber, sliced Kalamata olives, cherry tomatoes, and crumbled feta cheese should all be combined in a big bowl.
4. Mix the olive oil, red wine vinegar, dried oregano, salt, and pepper in a small bowl. After adding the dressing to the salad, toss to mix.
5. Separate the orzo salad into serving portions.
6. Let salad cool completely before freezing.

Grilled Eggplant and Hummus Wrap

Preparation Time: 20 minutes

Serves: 4

Calories: 300 **Sugar:** 5g **Sodium:** 450mg

Ingredients:

1 medium-sized eggplant, sliced

1 cup hummus

4 whole wheat wraps

1 cup cherry tomatoes, halved

1/2 cup cucumber, thinly sliced

1/4 cup red onion, thinly sliced

Fresh parsley, chopped

Olive oil

Salt and pepper to taste

Method of Preparation:

1. Drizzle slices of eggplant with olive oil and season with salt and pepper.
2. Grill for 3–4 minutes on each side, or until tender and slightly seared.
3. On each wrap, generously spread a layer of hummus.
4. Top the wraps with the grilled eggplant slices.
5. Evenly distribute the red onion, cucumber, and cherry tomatoes.
6. Add some fresh parsley on top.

7. Each wrapper should be carefully rolled, then toothpick-secured.

Freeze for later:

1. After cooking the meal, allow it to cool off.
2. Collect all the necessary supplies, such as; freezer-safe containers or bags, labels and a waterproof marker, plastic wrap or aluminum foil, Freezer tape (optional) and airtight vacuum sealer (optional)
3. Divide the meals into 4 containers or bags.
4. Clearly label each container or bag with the name of the dish, date of preparation, and any reheating instructions.
5. Lay bags flat in the freezer for quicker freezing and easy stacking. For containers, leave some space at the top to accommodate expansion during freezing.
6. Use older meals before newer ones to ensure nothing goes to waste.
7. Thaw and Reheat Safely

Tomato and Basil Bruschetta with Grilled Chicken

Preparation Time: 25 minutes

Serves: 4

Calories: 350 **Sugar:** 3g **Sodium:** 400mg

Ingredients:

4 boneless, skinless chicken breasts

1 cup cherry tomatoes, diced

1/2 cup fresh basil, chopped

2 cloves garlic, minced

2 tablespoons balsamic vinegar

2 tablespoons olive oil

Salt and pepper to taste

Baguette slices (for serving)

Method of Preparation:

1. Add salt and pepper to chicken breasts for seasoning.

2. Grill for 6 to 8 minutes on each side, or until well cooked.

3. Diced tomatoes, garlic, basil, olive oil, vinegar, and salt and pepper should all be combined in a bowl.

4. After giving the grilled chicken a few minutes to rest, cut it into thin strips.

5. Top each slice of baguette with a couple grilled chicken slices.

6. Add a dollop of tomato and basil bruschetta on top.

Freeze for later:

1. After cooking the meal, allow it to cool off.

2. Collect all the necessary supplies, such as; freezer-safe containers or bags, labels and a waterproof marker, plastic wrap or aluminum foil, Freezer tape (optional) and airtight vacuum sealer (optional)

3. Divide the meals into 4 containers or bags.

4. Clearly label each container or bag with the name of the dish, date of preparation, and any reheating instructions.

5. Lay bags flat in the freezer for quicker freezing and easy stacking. For containers, leave some space at the top to accommodate expansion during freezing.

6. Use older meals before newer ones to ensure nothing goes to waste.

7. Thaw and Reheat Safely

Spinach and Feta Stuffed Bell Peppers

Preparation Time: 40 minutes

Serves: 8

Calories: 400 **Sugar:** 5g **Sodium:** 350mg

Ingredients:

4 large bell peppers, halved and seeds removed

2 cups cooked quinoa

2 cups fresh spinach, chopped

1 cup feta cheese, crumbled

1 cup cherry tomatoes, diced

1/4 cup pine nuts

2 cloves garlic, minced

1 tablespoon olive oil

Salt and pepper to taste

Method of Preparation:

1. Turn the oven on to 375°F, or 190°C.
2. Cooked quinoa, spinach, feta cheese, cherry tomatoes, pine nuts, minced garlic, olive oil, salt, and pepper should all be combined in a big bowl.
3. Tightly pack the quinoa and spinach mixture into each side of the bell pepper.
4. Stuffed peppers should be baked for 25 to 30 minutes, or until they are soft, in a baking dish.

Freeze for later:

1. After cooking the meal, allow it to cool off.
2. Collect all the necessary supplies, such as; freezer-safe containers or bags, labels and a waterproof marker, plastic wrap or aluminum foil, Freezer tape (optional) and airtight vacuum sealer (optional)
3. Divide the meals into 8 containers or bags.
4. Clearly label each container or bag with the name of the dish, date of preparation, and any reheating instructions.

5. Lay bags flat in the freezer for quicker freezing and easy stacking. For containers, leave some space at the top to accommodate expansion during freezing.

6. Use older meals before newer ones to ensure nothing goes to waste.

7. Thaw and Reheat Safely

Greek Salad with Grilled Chicken

Preparation Time: 30 minutes

Serves: 4

Calories: 400 **Sugar:** 4g **Sodium:** 600mg

Ingredients:

1-pound boneless, skinless chicken breasts

2 tablespoons olive oil

1 teaspoon dried oregano

Salt and pepper to taste

1 large cucumber, diced

1 cup cherry tomatoes, halved

1 red onion, thinly sliced

1 cup Kalamata olives, pitted

1 cup feta cheese, crumbled

1/4 cup extra-virgin olive oil

2 tablespoons red wine vinegar

1 teaspoon dried oregano

Method of Preparation:

1. Set the grill's temperature to medium-high.
2. Season the chicken breasts with salt, pepper, dried oregano, and olive oil.
3. Cook the chicken for 6 to 8 minutes on each side, or until it's thoroughly done.
4. After a few minutes of rest, cut the chicken into strips.
5. Combine cucumber, olives, red onion, cherry tomatoes, and feta cheese in a big bowl.
6. To make the dressing, combine the red wine vinegar, dried oregano, and extra virgin olive oil in a small bowl.
7. Toss gently, then add the grilled chicken to the salad and drizzle with the dressing.

8. Separate into serving amounts and place in containers that may be frozen.

Freeze for later:

1. After cooking the meal, allow it to cool off.
2. Collect all the necessary supplies, such as; freezer-safe containers or bags, labels and a waterproof marker, plastic wrap or aluminum foil, Freezer tape (optional) and airtight vacuum sealer (optional)
3. Divide the meals into 4 containers or bags.
4. Clearly label each container or bag with the name of the dish, date of preparation, and any reheating instructions.
5. Lay bags flat in the freezer for quicker freezing and easy stacking. For containers, leave some space at the top to accommodate expansion during freezing.
6. Use older meals before newer ones to ensure nothing goes to waste.
7. Thaw and Reheat Safely

Mediterranean Turkey and Vegetable Skewers

Preparation Time: 25 minutes

Serves: 4

Calories: 300 **Sugar:** 3g **Sodium:** 400mg

Ingredients:

1 pound turkey breast, cut into cubes

2 zucchinis, sliced

1 red bell pepper, cut into chunks

1 yellow bell pepper, cut into chunks

1 red onion, cut into wedges

1/4 cup olive oil

2 cloves garlic, minced

1 teaspoon dried oregano

Salt and pepper to taste

Method of Preparation:

1. Set the oven or grill to a medium-high temperature.

2. Bell peppers, red onion, zucchini, and turkey cubes should all be combined in a bowl.

3. To make the marinade, combine olive oil, minced garlic, dried oregano, salt, and pepper in a small bowl.

4. Alternately thread the veggies and the meat onto skewers.

5. Apply the marinade on the skewers.

6. The turkey should be cooked through after 10 to 15 minutes of grilling or baking, with periodic flipping of the skewers.

7. Let cool before transferring to freezer-safe jars.

Freeze for later:

1. After cooking the meal, allow it to cool off.

2. Collect all the necessary supplies, such as; freezer-safe containers or bags, labels and a waterproof marker, plastic wrap or aluminum foil, Freezer tape (optional) and airtight vacuum sealer (optional)

3. Divide the meals into 4 containers or bags.

4. Clearly label each container or bag with the name of the dish, date of preparation, and any reheating instructions.

5. Lay bags flat in the freezer for quicker freezing and easy stacking. For containers, leave some space at the top to accommodate expansion during freezing.

6. Use older meals before newer ones to ensure nothing goes to waste.

7. Thaw and Reheat Safely

Baked Zucchini and Tomato Casserole

Preparation Time: 40 minutes

Serves: 6

Calories: 180 **Sugar:** 5g **Sodium:** 250mg

Ingredients:

4 medium zucchinis, sliced

2 cups cherry tomatoes, halved

1 onion, thinly sliced

2 cloves garlic, minced

1/4 cup fresh basil, chopped

1/4 cup fresh parsley, chopped

1/2 cup grated Parmesan cheese

2 tablespoons olive oil

Salt and pepper to taste

Method of Preparation:

1. Turn the oven on to 375°F, or 190°C.
2. Zest, cherry tomatoes, onion, garlic, basil, parsley, Parmesan cheese, olive oil, salt, and pepper should all be combined in a big bowl.
3. Spoon the mixture into an ovenproof dish.
4. Bake for 25 to 30 minutes, or until the top is golden brown and the vegetables are soft.
5. Let cool completely before dividing into freezer-safe portions.

Freeze for later:

1. After cooking the meal, allow it to cool off.

2. Collect all the necessary supplies, such as; freezer-safe containers or bags, labels and a waterproof marker, plastic wrap or aluminum foil, Freezer tape (optional) and airtight vacuum sealer (optional)
3. Divide the meals into 6 containers or bags.
4. Clearly label each container or bag with the name of the dish, date of preparation, and any reheating instructions.
5. Lay bags flat in the freezer for quicker freezing and easy stacking. For containers, leave some space at the top to accommodate expansion during freezing.
6. Use older meals before newer ones to ensure nothing goes to waste.
7. Thaw and Reheat Safely

Olive and Herb Crusted Cod with Quinoa

Preparation Time: 30 minutes

Serves: 4

Calories: 250 **Sugar:** 1g **Sodium:** 400mg

Ingredients:

4 cod fillets

1/2 cup pitted Kalamata olives, chopped

2 tablespoons fresh parsley, chopped

1 tablespoon fresh oregano, chopped

2 tablespoons breadcrumbs

2 tablespoons olive oil

1 lemon, sliced

Salt and pepper to taste

2 cups cooked quinoa

Method of Preparation:

1. Set oven temperature to 400°F, or 200°C.
2. To make the crust, put the breadcrumbs, olive oil, salt, pepper, parsley, and chopped olives in a bowl.
3. Cod fillets should be placed on a parchment paper-lined baking pan.
4. Place a crust made of herbs and olives on top of every fish fillet.

5. Add slices of lemon on top.

6. Bake the cod for 15 to 20 minutes, or until the crust is golden brown and the fish is cooked through.

7. After cooking the quinoa, serve and let cool before freezing in individual servings.

Freeze for later:

1. After cooking the meal, allow it to cool off.

2. Collect all the necessary supplies, such as; freezer-safe containers or bags, labels and a waterproof marker, plastic wrap or aluminum foil, Freezer tape (optional) and airtight vacuum sealer (optional)

3. Divide the meals into 4 containers or bags.

4. Clearly label each container or bag with the name of the dish, date of preparation, and any reheating instructions.

5. Lay bags flat in the freezer for quicker freezing and easy stacking. For containers, leave some space at the top to accommodate expansion during freezing.

6. Use older meals before newer ones to ensure nothing goes to waste.

7. Thaw and Reheat Safely

DINNER

Baked Mediterranean Chicken with Lemon and Olives

Preparation Time: 45 minutes

Serves: 4 Serves

Calories: 350 **Sugar:** 1g **Sodium:** 600mg

Ingredients:

4 boneless, skinless chicken breasts

1/4 cup extra-virgin olive oil

2 lemons (1 juiced and zested, 1 sliced)

1 cup pitted Kalamata olive

4 cloves garlic, minced

1 teaspoon dried oregano

1 teaspoon dried thyme

Salt and pepper to taste

Method of Preparation:

1. Turn the oven on to 375°F, or 190°C.

2. Mix the olive oil, lemon zest, juice, minced garlic, oregano, thyme, salt, and pepper in a small bowl.

3. Transfer the chicken breasts to a baking dish and cover them with the lemon-olive oil mixture.

4. Transfer the olives and lemon slices to the baking dish.

5. Bake the chicken for 25 to 30 minutes, or until it is cooked through, in a preheated oven.

6. Warm up and savor!

Freeze for later:

1. After cooking the meal, allow it to cool off.

2. Collect all the necessary supplies, such as; freezer-safe containers or bags, labels and a waterproof marker, plastic wrap or aluminum foil, Freezer tape (optional) and airtight vacuum sealer (optional)

3. Divide the meals into 4 containers or bags.

4. Clearly label each container or bag with the name of the dish, date of preparation, and any reheating instructions.

5. Lay bags flat in the freezer for quicker freezing and easy stacking. For containers, leave some space at the top to accommodate expansion during freezing.
6. Use older meals before newer ones to ensure nothing goes to waste.
7. Thaw and Reheat Safely

Lemon Herb Quinoa with Roasted Vegetables

Preparation Time: 45 minutes

Serves: 4

Calories: 280 **Sugar:** 4g **Sodium:** 300mg

Ingredients:

1 cup quinoa, rinsed

2 cups water or vegetable broth

2 tablespoons olive oil

1 lemon (juiced and zested)

1 teaspoon dried thyme

1 teaspoon dried rosemary

Salt and pepper to taste

Assorted vegetables (e.g., cherry tomatoes, zucchini, bell peppers), chopped

Method of Preparation:

1. Set oven temperature to 400°F, or 200°C.
2. Quinoa should be combined with water or vegetable broth in a saucepan.
3. After bringing to a boil, lower the heat, cover, and simmer the quinoa for 15 minutes, or until it is tender.
4. Combine chopped veggies with salt, pepper, thyme, rosemary, lemon juice, and olive oil.
5. Arrange the veggies onto a baking sheet and bake for 20 to 25 minutes in an oven that has been preheated.
6. Using a fork, fluff the cooked quinoa and mix it with the roasted veggies.
7. Serve heated as a light main course or as a side dish.

Freeze for later:

1. After cooking the meal, allow it to cool off.
2. Collect all the necessary supplies, such as; freezer-safe containers or bags, labels and a waterproof

marker, plastic wrap or aluminum foil, Freezer tape (optional) and airtight vacuum sealer (optional)

3. Divide the meals into 4 containers or bags.
4. Clearly label each container or bag with the name of the dish, date of preparation, and any reheating instructions.
5. Lay bags flat in the freezer for quicker freezing and easy stacking. For containers, leave some space at the top to accommodate expansion during freezing.
6. Use older meals before newer ones to ensure nothing goes to waste.
7. Thaw and Reheat Safely

Mediterranean Shrimp and Tomato Skewers

Preparation Time: 35 minutes

Serves: 4 Serves

Calories: 220 **Sugar:** 2g **Sodium:** 400mg

Ingredients:

1-pound large shrimp, peeled and deveined

1-pint cherry tomatoes

1/4 cup extra-virgin olive oil

2 cloves garlic, minced

1 teaspoon dried oregano

1 teaspoon smoked paprika

Salt and pepper to taste

Wooden skewers, soaked in water

Method of Preparation:

1. Turn the heat up to medium-high on the grill or grill pan.
2. Combine olive oil, smoked paprika, oregano, minced garlic, salt, and pepper in a bowl.
3. Cherry tomatoes and shrimp should be alternately threaded onto moistened wooden skewers.
4. Apply the olive oil mixture to the skewers.
5. Cook the shrimp on the skewers for 3–4 minutes on each side, or until they are thoroughly done.
6. Savor the tastes of the Mediterranean while serving hot!

Freeze for later:

1. After cooking the meal, allow it to cool off.

2. Collect all the necessary supplies, such as; freezer-safe containers or bags, labels and a waterproof marker, plastic wrap or aluminum foil, Freezer tape (optional) and airtight vacuum sealer (optional)

3. Divide the meals into 4 containers or bags.

4. Clearly label each container or bag with the name of the dish, date of preparation, and any reheating instructions.

5. Lay bags flat in the freezer for quicker freezing and easy stacking. For containers, leave some space at the top to accommodate expansion during freezing.

6. Use older meals before newer ones to ensure nothing goes to waste.

7. Thaw and Reheat Safely

Greek Lamb Meatballs with Mint Yogurt Sauce

Preparation Time: 30 minutes

Serves: 4

Calories: 350 **Sugar:** 2g **Sodium:** 450mg

Ingredients:

1 lb. ground lamb

1/2 cup breadcrumbs

1/4 cup finely chopped red onion

2 cloves garlic, minced

1 tsp dried oregano

1 tsp ground cumin

Salt and pepper to taste

1 egg, beaten

Olive oil for cooking

Mint Yogurt Sauce:

1 cup Greek yogurt

2 tbsp fresh mint, finely chopped

1 tbsp lemon juice

Salt to taste

Method of Preparation:

1. Ground lamb, breadcrumbs, red onion, garlic, oregano, cumin, salt, pepper, and beaten egg should all be combined in a big bowl.
2. Blend thoroughly.
3. Form the ingredients into meatballs with a diameter of roughly one inch.
4. In a skillet over medium heat, warm the olive oil.
5. Cook the meatballs until they are well cooked and browned on all sides.
6. In a bowl, combine Greek yogurt, mint, lemon juice, and salt to make the mint yogurt sauce.
7. Present the meatballs alongside the mint yogurt sauce.

Freeze for later:

1. After cooking the meal, allow it to cool off.
2. Collect all the necessary supplies, such as; freezer-safe containers or bags, labels and a waterproof marker, plastic wrap or aluminum foil, Freezer tape (optional) and airtight vacuum sealer (optional)
3. Divide the meals into 4 containers or bags.

4. Clearly label each container or bag with the name of the dish, date of preparation, and any reheating instructions.

5. Lay bags flat in the freezer for quicker freezing and easy stacking. For containers, leave some space at the top to accommodate expansion during freezing.

6. Use older meals before newer ones to ensure nothing goes to waste.

7. Thaw and Reheat Safely

Roasted Eggplant and Chickpea Stew

Preparation Time: 45 minutes

Serves: 6

Calories: 250 **Sugar:** 5g **Sodium:** 600mg

Ingredients:

1 large eggplant, diced

1 can (15 oz) chickpeas, drained and rinsed

1 onion, finely chopped

3 cloves garlic, minced

1 can (14 oz) diced tomatoes

1 tsp cumin

1 tsp smoked paprika

Salt and pepper to taste

Olive oil for roasting

Method of Preparation:

1. Set oven temperature to 400°F, or 200°C.
2. After putting chopped eggplant on a baking sheet and tossing it in olive oil, roast it for 20 to 25 minutes, or until it turns golden brown.
3. Add the garlic and onions to a large pot and sauté until softened.
4. Stir in the diced tomatoes, cumin, smoked paprika, salt, and pepper.
5. Add the chickpeas.
6. After adding the roasted eggplant, boil the stew for fifteen to twenty minutes.

Freeze for later:

1. After cooking the meal, allow it to cool off.

2. Collect all the necessary supplies, such as; freezer-safe containers or bags, labels and a waterproof marker, plastic wrap or aluminum foil, Freezer tape (optional) and airtight vacuum sealer (optional)

3. Divide the meals into 6 containers or bags.

4. Clearly label each container or bag with the name of the dish, date of preparation, and any reheating instructions.

5. Lay bags flat in the freezer for quicker freezing and easy stacking. For containers, leave some space at the top to accommodate expansion during freezing.

6. Use older meals before newer ones to ensure nothing goes to waste.

7. Thaw and Reheat Safely

Tomato Basil Cod Fillets

Preparation Time: 25 minutes

Serves: 4

Calories: 200 **Sugar:** 3g **Sodium:** 300mg

Ingredients:

4 cod fillets

2 cups cherry tomatoes, halved

3 tbsp olive oil

3 cloves garlic, minced

1/4 cup fresh basil, chopped

Salt and pepper to taste

Lemon wedges for serving

Method of Preparation:

1. Turn the oven on to 375°F, or 190°C.
2. Cod fillets should be put on a baking dish.
3. Add a dash of olive oil and season with salt and pepper.
4. Add fresh basil, minced garlic, and cherry tomatoes to a bowl.
5. Over the fish fillets, spoon mixture.
6. Bake the fish for 15 to 20 minutes, or until it is well done.
7. Accompany with wedges of lemon.

Freeze for later:

1. After cooking the meal, allow it to cool off.

2. Collect all the necessary supplies, such as; freezer-safe containers or bags, labels and a waterproof marker, plastic wrap or aluminum foil, Freezer tape (optional) and airtight vacuum sealer (optional)
3. Divide the meals into 4 containers or bags.
4. Clearly label each container or bag with the name of the dish, date of preparation, and any reheating instructions.
5. Lay bags flat in the freezer for quicker freezing and easy stacking. For containers, leave some space at the top to accommodate expansion during freezing.
6. Use older meals before newer ones to ensure nothing goes to waste.
7. Thaw and Reheat Safely

Mediterranean Turkey and Zucchini Patties

Preparation Time: 30 minutes

Serves: 4

Calories: 250 **Sugar:** 1g **Sodium:** 300mg

Ingredients:

1 pound ground turkey

2 medium-sized zucchinis, grated and drained

1/2 cup breadcrumbs

1/4 cup feta cheese, crumbled

1/4 cup fresh parsley, chopped

1 teaspoon dried oregano

Salt and pepper to taste

Olive oil for cooking

Method of Preparation:

1. Ground turkey, shredded and drained zucchini, breadcrumbs, feta cheese, chopped parsley, dried oregano, salt, and pepper should all be combined in a big mixing basin.
2. After thoroughly combining the ingredients, shape the dough into patties of the required size.
3. In a skillet over medium heat, warm the olive oil.

4. Cook the patties until they are cooked through and have a golden-brown color, about 5 to 7 minutes on each side.

5. After letting the patties cool, cover each one separately in plastic wrap and store in a freezer-safe container.

6. After adding the date to the container, freeze it.

Freeze for later:

1. After cooking the meal, allow it to cool off.

2. Collect all the necessary supplies, such as; freezer-safe containers or bags, labels and a waterproof marker, plastic wrap or aluminum foil, Freezer tape (optional) and airtight vacuum sealer (optional)

3. Divide the meals into 2 containers or bags.

4. Clearly label each container or bag with the name of the dish, date of preparation, and any reheating instructions.

5. Lay bags flat in the freezer for quicker freezing and easy stacking. For containers, leave some space at the top to accommodate expansion during freezing.

6. Use older meals before newer ones to ensure nothing goes to waste.

7. Thaw and Reheat Safely

Freeze for later:

1. After cooking the meal, allow it to cool off.

2. Collect all the necessary supplies, such as; freezer-safe containers or bags, labels and a waterproof marker, plastic wrap or aluminum foil, Freezer tape (optional) and airtight vacuum sealer (optional)

3. Divide the meals into 4 containers or bags.

4. Clearly label each container or bag with the name of the dish, date of preparation, and any reheating instructions.

5. Lay bags flat in the freezer for quicker freezing and easy stacking. For containers, leave some space at the top to accommodate expansion during freezing.

6. Use older meals before newer ones to ensure nothing goes to waste.

7. Thaw and Reheat Safely

Quinoa Tabbouleh with Cucumber and Cherry Tomatoes

Preparation Time: 30 minutes

Serves: 4

Calories: 300 **Sugar:** 2g **Sodium:** 150mg

Ingredients:

1 cup quinoa, rinsed

2 cups water

1 cucumber, diced

1 cup cherry tomatoes, halved

1/2 cup fresh parsley, chopped

1/4 cup fresh mint, chopped

1/4 cup red onion, finely chopped

1/4 cup olive oil

2 tablespoons lemon juice

Salt and pepper to taste

Method of Preparation:

1. Quinoa and water should be combined in a medium pot.

2. After bringing to a boil, lower heat, cover, and simmer the quinoa for fifteen minutes, or until it is tender and the water has been absorbed.

3. Using a fork, fluff the quinoa and allow it to come to room temperature.

4. The cooked quinoa, cucumber, cherry tomatoes, parsley, mint, and red onion should all be combined in a big bowl.

5. Mix the olive oil, lemon juice, salt, and pepper in a small bowl. Drizzle the quinoa mixture over top and mix thoroughly.

6. After letting the tabbouleh cool, pour it into freezer-safe containers, making sure to leave room at the top.

7. Once the containers are frozen, mark them with the date.

Freeze for later:

1. After cooking the meal, allow it to cool off.

2. Collect all the necessary supplies, such as; freezer-safe containers or bags, labels and a waterproof marker, plastic wrap or aluminum foil, Freezer tape (optional) and airtight vacuum sealer (optional)

3. Divide the meals into 4 containers or bags.

4. Clearly label each container or bag with the name of the dish, date of preparation, and any reheating instructions.

5. Lay bags flat in the freezer for quicker freezing and easy stacking. For containers, leave some space at the top to accommodate expansion during freezing.

6. Use older meals before newer ones to ensure nothing goes to waste.

7. Thaw and Reheat Safely

Greek Style Stuffed Peppers with Ground Turkey

Preparation Time: 45 minutes

Serves: 4

Calories: 350 **Sugar:** 4g **Sodium:** 400mg

Ingredients:

4 large bell peppers, halved and seeds removed

1 pound ground turkey

1 cup cooked brown rice

1 can (14 oz) diced tomatoes, drained

1/2 cup feta cheese, crumbled

1/4 cup Kalamata olives, chopped

1/4 cup fresh parsley, chopped

1 teaspoon dried oregano

Salt and pepper to taste

Olive oil for drizzling

Method of Preparation:

1. Turn the oven on to 375°F, or 190°C.
2. Cook the ground turkey in a pan until browned. Remove any extra fat.
3. The cooked turkey, brown rice, diced tomatoes, feta cheese, dried oregano, Kalamata olives, parsley, and salt and pepper should all be combined in a big bowl.
4. Stuff the bell pepper halves with the turkey mixture and place them in a baking tray.
5. After brushing the filled peppers with olive oil, cover the baking dish with foil.
6. Bake peppers for 25 to 30 minutes, or until soft.

7. After the filled peppers have cooled, move them to freezer-safe containers.

8. Once the containers are frozen, mark them with the date.

Freeze for later:

1. After cooking the meal, allow it to cool off.

2. Collect all the necessary supplies, such as; freezer-safe containers or bags, labels and a waterproof marker, plastic wrap or aluminum foil, Freezer tape (optional) and airtight vacuum sealer (optional)

3. Divide the meals into 4 containers or bags.

4. Clearly label each container or bag with the name of the dish, date of preparation, and any reheating instructions.

5. Lay bags flat in the freezer for quicker freezing and easy stacking. For containers, leave some space at the top to accommodate expansion during freezing.

6. Use older meals before newer ones to ensure nothing goes to waste.

7. Thaw and Reheat Safely

Chickpea and Spinach Curry with Couscous

Preparation Time: 40 minutes

Serves: 4

Calories: 400 **Sugar:** 5g **Sodium:** 500mg

Ingredients:

1 can (15 oz) chickpeas, drained and rinsed

1 onion, finely chopped

2 cloves garlic, minced

1 tablespoon curry powder

1 teaspoon ground cumin

1 teaspoon ground coriander

1 can (14 oz) diced tomatoes

1 can (14 oz) coconut milk

4 cups fresh spinach

Salt and pepper to taste

2 cups cooked couscous

Method of Preparation:

1. Minced garlic and diced onion should be sautéed in a big skillet until they are tender.
2. Cook for a further one to two minutes after adding the curry powder, ground cumin, and ground coriander to the skillet.
3. Add the diced tomatoes, coconut milk, and chickpeas.
4. Simmer, stirring often, for 15 to 20 minutes.
5. Cook the fresh spinach in the skillet until it wilts.
6. Add salt and pepper to taste when preparing the curry.
7. After letting the curry cool, divide it into freezer-safe portions.
8. After cooked, transfer couscous to different containers.
9. Once the containers are frozen, mark them with the date.

Freeze for later:

1. After cooking the meal, allow it to cool off.

2. Collect all the necessary supplies, such as; freezer-safe containers or bags, labels and a waterproof marker, plastic wrap or aluminum foil, Freezer tape (optional) and airtight vacuum sealer (optional)

3. Divide the meals into 4 containers or bags.

4. Clearly label each container or bag with the name of the dish, date of preparation, and any reheating instructions.

5. Lay bags flat in the freezer for quicker freezing and easy stacking. For containers, leave some space at the top to accommodate expansion during freezing.

6. Use older meals before newer ones to ensure nothing goes to waste.

7. Thaw and Reheat Safely

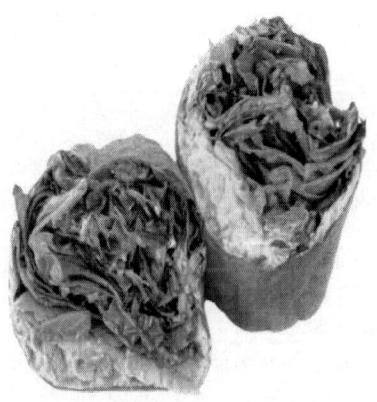

CONCLUSION

To sum up, this book is a culinary adventure that will change the way you prepare meals and improve your ability to eat healthily and flavorfully.

By the time you finish this cookbook, you will have a newfound appreciation for the wide variety and depth of flavors found throughout the Mediterranean region.

You have accepted the health advantages of the Mediterranean diet in addition to learning how simple it is to prepare delectable meals ahead of time thanks to the well-chosen recipes in this book.

You've been able to make healthier decisions without sacrificing flavor or nutrition thanks to the marriage of colorful, fresh ingredients and the ease of freezer-friendly recipes.

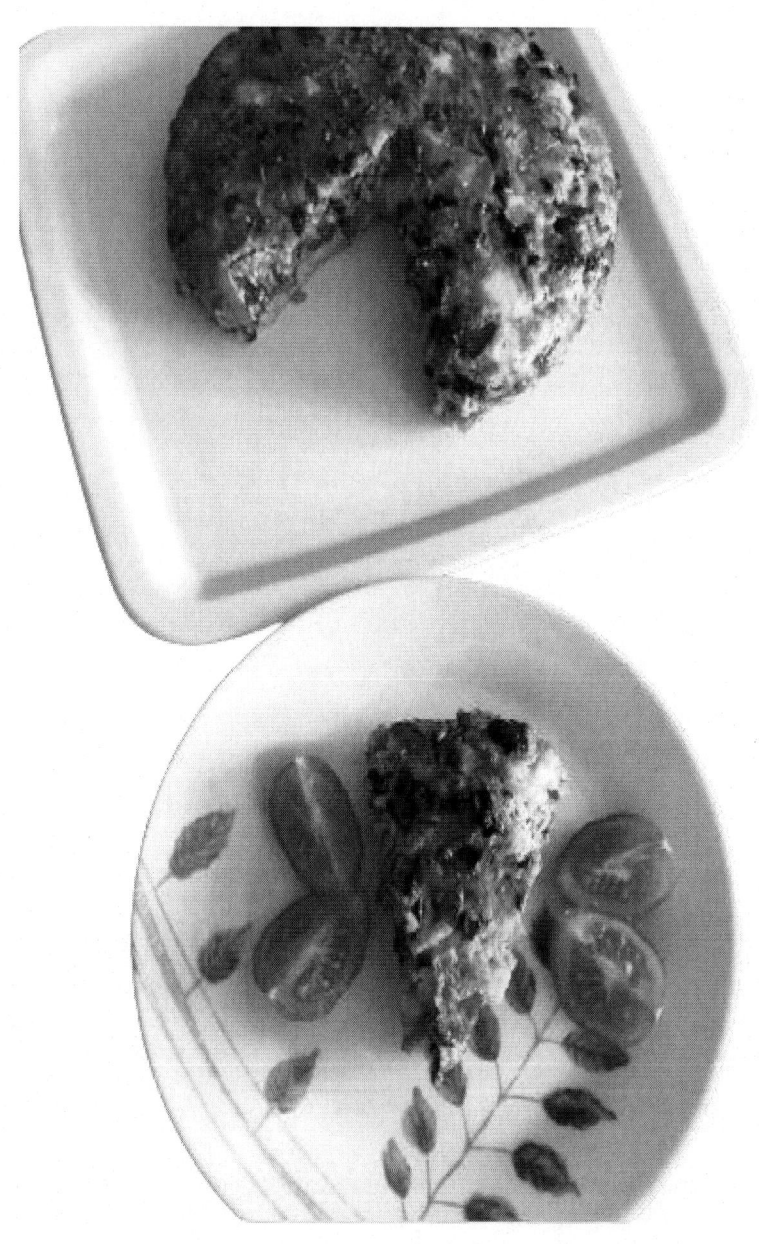

13492535R00055